Easy, Healthy & Flavorful

The cookbook for weight loss, weight management and everyday healthy eating.

Nutri Health & Body Company

About the Author

As far as I can remember I have always been
fascinated by food and cooking. Growing up I
would always help my Mom with recipes or just
watch in awe waiting til that one day when I
could cook.

Fast forward to being a teenager living on her
own and having no choice but to learn how to
cook. Through the years I got better and better,
until I realized I had a true passion and talent
for it.

Before I knew it, I started developing my own
healthy recipes to help me lose weight.

Fast forward again to 2017 when I publish my
first cookbook! I have never been happier waking
up doing what I love everyday and making people
happy with my food and even better, helping
people live a healthier lifestyle. I will never
turn back.

I chose the Nutri-tious life and I hope you do too.
Bon appetit!

Chicken Salad

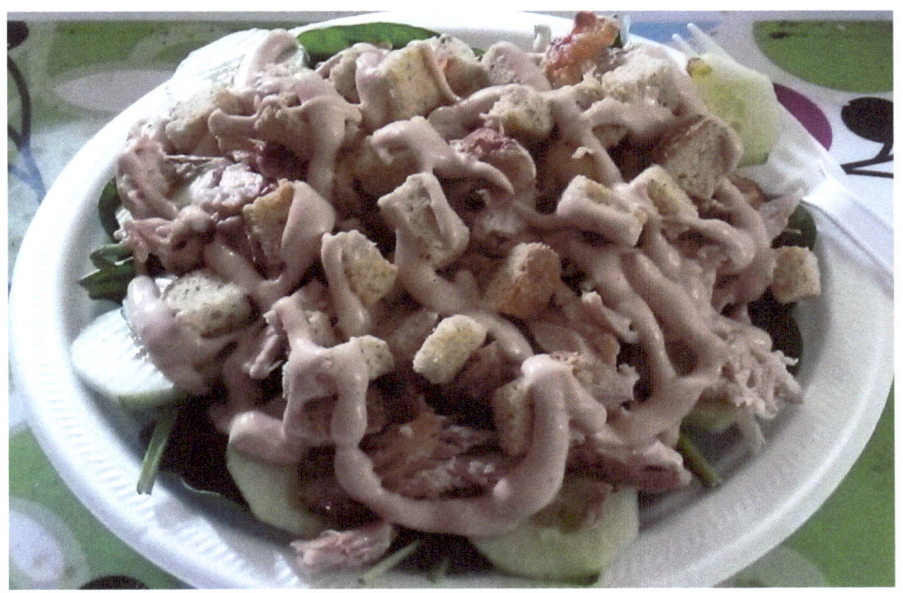

This is my favourite salad to make. It's very nutritious and gives you your full serving of veggies for the day. This is very filling and great for lunch or dinner.

You will need:
- **Cooked chicken breast** (air fried or oven baked)
- **Veggies** (cucumbers or bell peppers of any colour)
- **Baby Spinach** (fresh)
- **Dressing** (all natural ranch or all natural romano caesar)
- **Croutons** (Rye bread croutons or desired flavor)
- **Himalayan Pink Salt** (few pinches)
- **Black pepper** (few pinches)
- **Parsley** (few pinches)

First lay a bed of spinach onto a plate. Next chop up your veggies and place them on top of the spinach. Chop up your cooked chicken and place it on top of the veggies. Place your croutons on top of the veggies. Add dressing and seasonings, then grab a fork and enjoy! Bon appetit!

Nutri Tip: This salad is spectacular paired with a fruity red wine.

Chicken Fried Rice

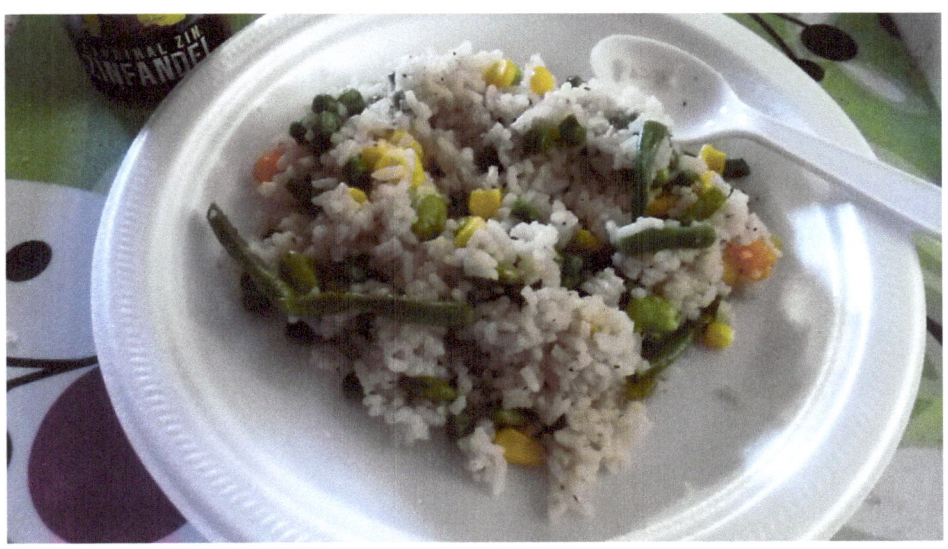

I love making this rice! It's so easy, so flavorful and so healthy. You only need 3 ingredients so it's even cheap to make. Like I always say, eating healthy doesn't have to be expensive.

You will need:
- **Frozen Veggies** (any blend of your choice)
- **Instant Rice** (4 cups, cooked)
- **Chicken Broth** (450ml)
- **Chicken** (cooked, quartered)
- **Rainbow Peppercorn Medley** (desired amount)
- **Garlic Powder** (desired amount)

Heat frying pan on medium. Throw in cooked rice then add chicken broth. Add desired amount of frozen veggies and cooked chicken. Reduce heat to simmer. Add seasonings if desired and let simmer until all the broth has soaked into the rice. Stir occasionally. Turn off heat and it's ready to plate. Bon Appetit!

Nutri Tip: I love making big batches of this for leftovers. Next time I want to eat it, I warm it up in the frying pan again and add more broth til it soaks into the rice. It gets more and more flavorful every time I make it!

BBQ Chicken Tostadas

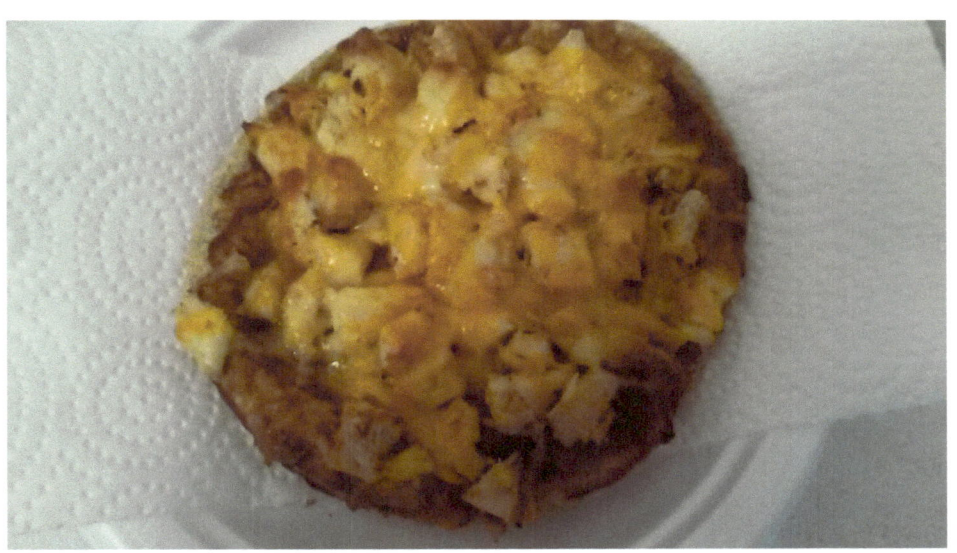

These are one of my favourite snacks to make in the summer because they cook fast and are delicious!

You will need:
- **Cooked Chicken** (cooked, quartered, baked or air fried)
- **Mozzarella Cheese** (shredded)
- **Pita Bread** (whole wheat)
- **BBQ Sauce** (desired brand)

Optional:
- **Bell Peppers** (orange)

Preheat your oven to 425 degrees Fahrenheit. Spread barbecue sauce onto the pita bread. Put on desired amount of chicken then sprinkle on desired amount of shredded cheese. Place in oven directly on rack for 2 minutes. Turn off oven and place on broil for 2 minutes or until cheese melted. Use tongs to transfer to plate. Bon Appetit!

Nutri Tip: These are easy to make with canned tuna as well instead of chicken! Just substitute BBQ sauce for Dijon mustard.

Mexican Dip

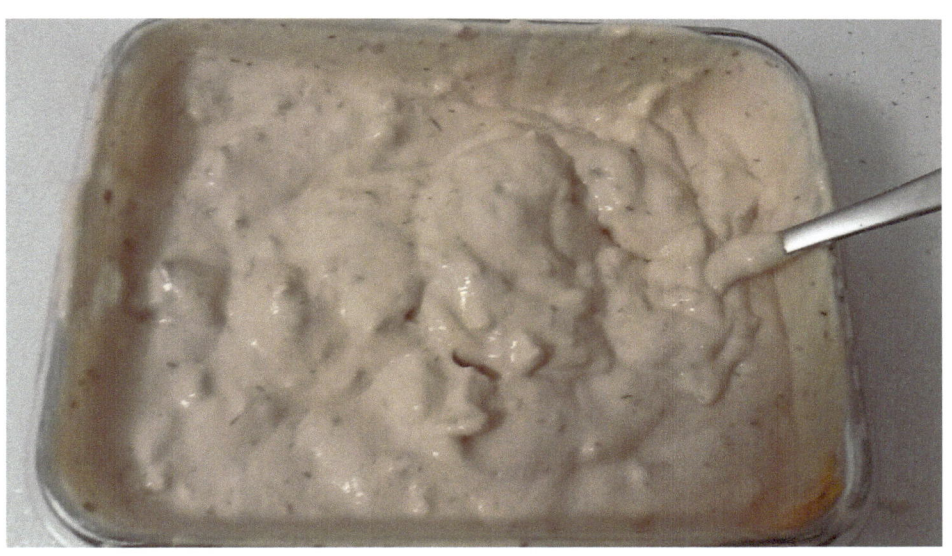

This is an easy, flavorful dip you can pretty much dip anything in!

You will need:
- **Sour Cream** (500ml, 14% M.F.)
- **Dill weed** (1tsp-1tbsp, add to taste)
- **Salsa** (1 cup of mild or spicy)
- **Dehydrated Jalapeno Flakes** (few pinches)
- **Crushed Red Pepper Flakes** (few pinches)
- **Garlic Powder** (few pinches)
- **Shredded Cheese** (1 cup, any cheese of your choice)

Grab a medium sized container. Scoop in the sour cream and salsa. Sprinkle in all the seasonings except for the dill weed. Stir and gradually sprinkle in dill weed. Add shredded cheese and stir until completely blended. Pair with your snack of choice. Bon appetit!

Nutri Tip: You can use any cheese you like but my favourites to use are mozzarella, monterey jack or a tex mex mix. This also stores in the fridge for up to 4 days.

Holubtsi/Lazy Man's Cabbage Rolls

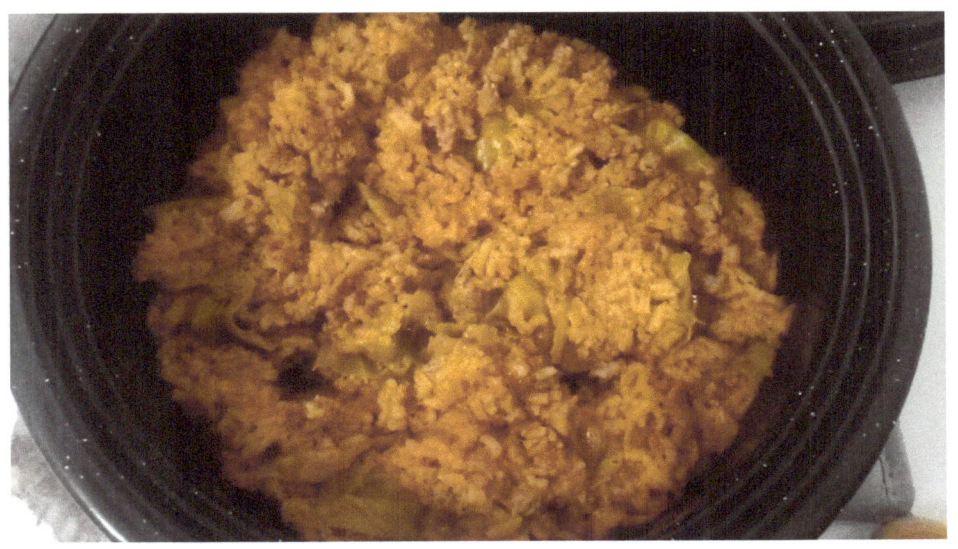

Cabbage rolls we're always my favourite Ukrainian dish growing up, but this is my lazier, healthier twist on it!

You will need:
- **Ground turkey** (1 lb, browned)
- **Fresh cabbage** (4 cups or 4-5 large leaves)
- **Tomato soup** (1 can)
- **Instant Rice** (1 cup, uncooked)
- **Rainbow Peppercorn Medley** (desired amount)
- **Garlic Powder** (desired amount)
- **Garlic Salt** (a pinch)

First preheat your oven to 350 degrees Fahrenheit. In a frying pan, brown ground turkey. Next wash, rinse and chop cabbage. Grab a large roasting pot and put your first layer of cabbage loosely along the bottom of the pan.

Next grab a large bowl and pour in ground turkey, rice and seasonings then stir until completely mixed. Add a layer of the mixture on top of the cabbage in roasting pot, then add a layer of cabbage on top of mixture. Continue so on and so forth until all cabbage and ground turkey is used.

Prepare canned tomato soup as directed on can and simmer until no longer chunky. Once tomato soup is done, pour over top of your layers.

Lastly throw it in the oven for 1 ½ hours – 2 hours depending on your oven. Stir every 45 minutes so it doesn't dry out. When your cabbage is soft and the rice is cooked, it's ready! Bon appetit!

Lazy Stuffed Chicken

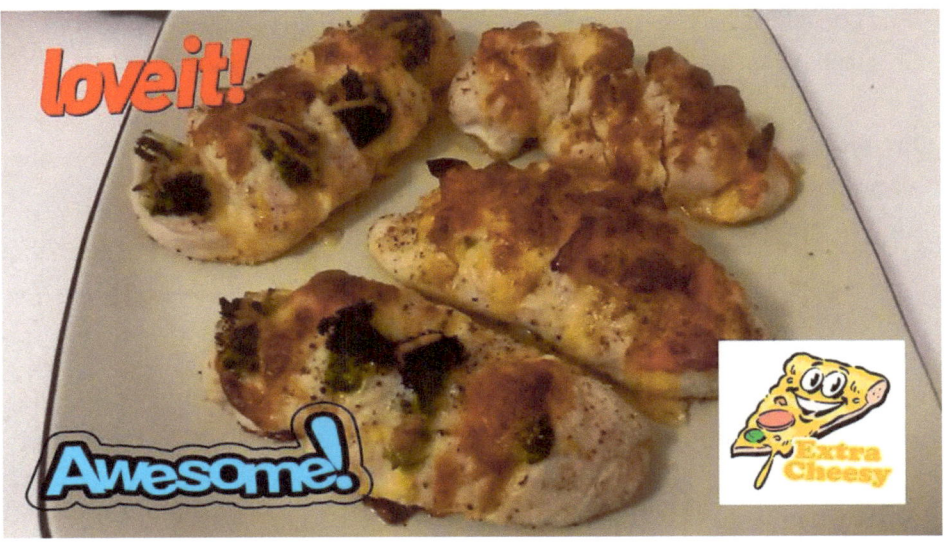

Who doesn't love a good stuffed chicken?
Well this one is a lot easier to make
and if I may say, so much more
delicious!

You will need:
- **Broccoli** (frozen or fresh)
- **Bell Peppers** (Orange or any desired colour)
- **Mozzarella Cheese** (shredded)
- **Chicken Breast** (boneless, skinless, raw)(the plumper the better)

Optional:
- Himalayan Pink Salt
- Black Pepper

First preheat your oven to 400 degrees Fahrenheit. Grab chicken breasts, place horizontally and cut vertical slits deep, but not all the way through. Make sure the slits aren't too close together (4-5 slits).
Next stuff the slits half way with cheese then stuff the rest with broccoli/peppers. You can sprinkle cheese on top of the stuffed chicken, if desired (it also helps keep the veggies in). Now throw it in the oven for 30 minutes or until chicken is completely cooked. Bon Appetit!

Nutri Tip: This is great paired with any type of fresh salad and a medium-bodied red wine.

Goat Cheese Grilled Cheese

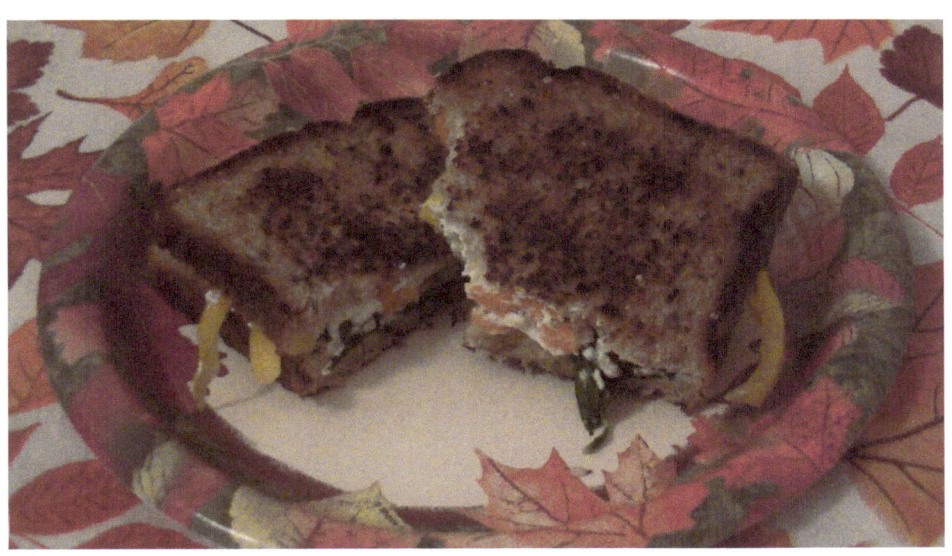

When you're trying to lose weight, who says you can't have a grilled cheese? This one is so flavorful and so crispy, it's pure heaven. You will never go back to that plain old grilled cheese!

You will need:
- **Goat cheese** (softened at room temperature)
- **Orange & Yellow Bell Peppers** (1 of each)
- **Whole Wheat Bread** (2 slices)
- **Coconut Oil** (1 tbsp)
- **Baby Spinach** (fresh)
- **Dijon Mustard** (desired amount)

First slice bell peppers into rings (4 rings per sandwich). Next spread desired amount of Dijon mustard on one slice of bread. On the other slice of bread, spread on desired amount of goat cheese. Place bell pepper rings on the goat cheese and spinach on Dijon mustard.

Grab a small frying pan and heat up the coconut oil on medium high heat. When oil is heated, place sandwich in frying pan. Fry your grilled cheese 2-3 minutes on each side or until cheese is melted and bread is cooked to your liking. Once it's done, time to plate and enjoy. So crispy! Bon appetit!

Nutri Tip: This grilled cheese can also be made in a panini maker/sandwich maker minus the coconut oil. You can switch up the veggies for variety as well. Also, this would be great paired with a fruity, light to medium-bodied red wine.

Slow Cooker Honey Pineapple Flat Ham

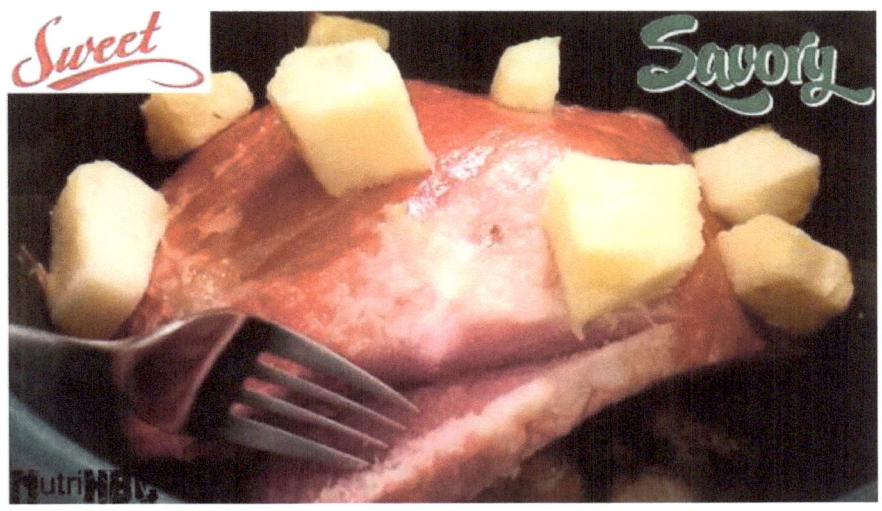

This ham is so easy and so flavorful, it literally speaks for itself! The perfect healthy recipe to make at Christmas time or Thanksgiving.

You will need:
-**Flat Ham** (pre-cooked, shoulder, hickory smoked)
-**Raw Honey** ($\frac{1}{4}$ cup)
-**Pineapple** ($\frac{1}{2}$ of 1 whole, fresh)

First cut pineapple into chunks and place half of the amount into bottom of slow cooker. Mash pineapple with a potato masher to extract the juice. This will act as a base for your ham. Place ham on top of the mashed pineapple then drizzle honey onto ham. Next place remaining pineapple chunks randomly on top of ham (the honey glaze will act like glue). Throw the lid on your slow cooker and set it on low for 4-6 hours. Once it's done, slice it up and enjoy! Bon appetit!

Nutri Tip: Slow cooking a ham makes it much more juicier and flavorful than cooking it in an oven, easier too!

Ham & Turkey Protein Bites

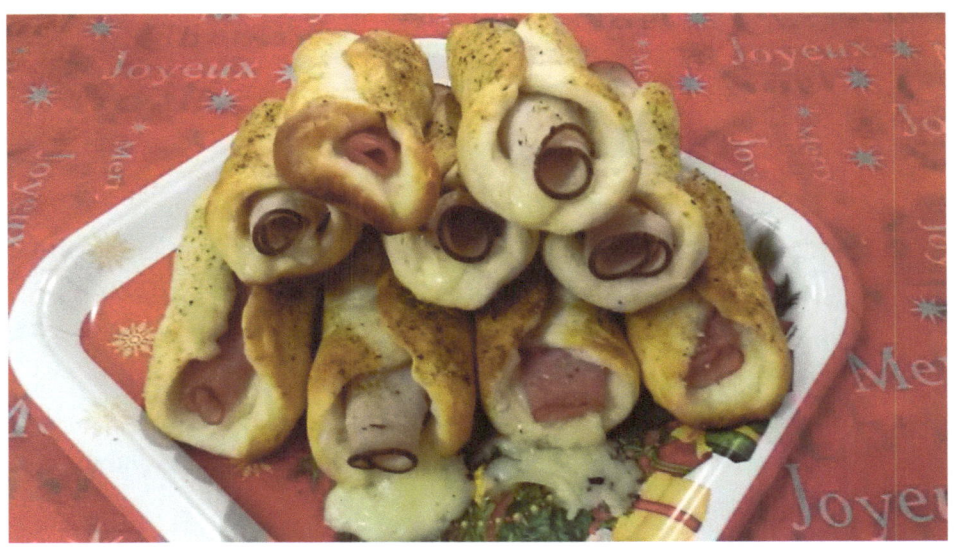

These are my favourite to snack on before/after a workout. A quick and easy way to get a protein boost!

You will need:
-**Ham** (5 slices, sliced lunch-meat style)
-**Turkey** (5 slices, sliced lunch-meat style)
-**Mozzarella Cheese** (10 slices)
-**Garlic & Herb Seasoning**
-**Dough** (pre-made biscuit dough, makes 10)

First preheat your oven to 400 degrees Fahrenheit. Flatten each piece of dough by hand about 4-5 inches wide and place on a baking sheet. Place one slice of cheese in the middle of each piece of dough. Roll each slice of turkey/ham and place on top of the cheese. Pull each side of the dough to meet each other and press together to seal them. You can also press along all sides of the dough to enclose the cheese. Sprinkle garlic & herb seasoning on top of bites.
Lastly, throw them in the oven for 10-15 minutes or until golden brown. Once they are done, let cool for 10 minutes and they are ready to eat. Bon appetit!

Nutri Tip: You could store these in a Ziploc bag in the fridge for up to a week! You can reheat them in the microwave for 10-15 seconds or broil in the oven on top rack for 2 minutes.

Peanut Butter Munch

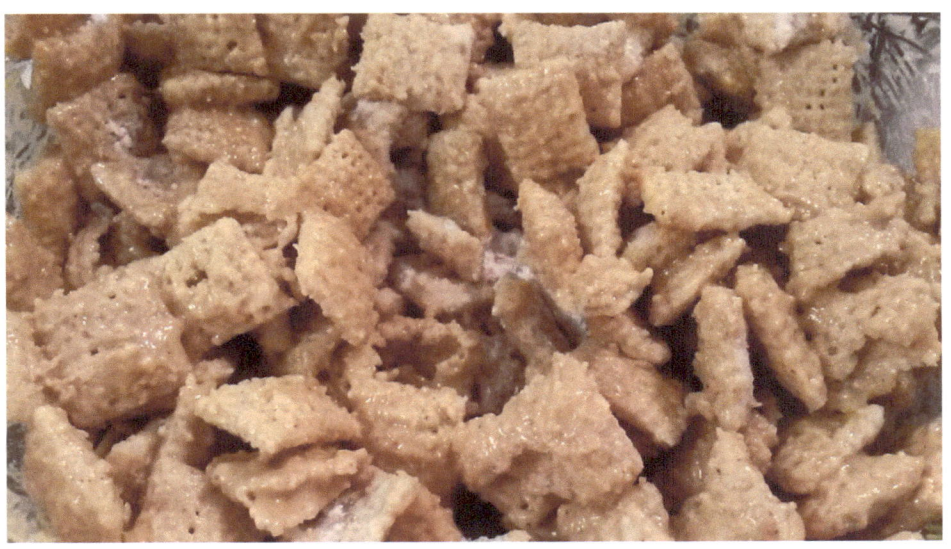

Anything peanut butter is an absolute favourite of mine, so this is a real treat. This is a snack that tastes naughty, but there's nothing to be guilty about.....it's all healthy ingredients!

You will need:
-**Chex** (3 cups, Rice or Corn)
-**Raw Honey** ($\frac{1}{4}$ cup)
-**All Natural Peanut Butter** ($\frac{1}{2}$ cup)
-**Icing Sugar** ($\frac{1}{4}$ cup or desired amount)

First pour the Chex into a medium sized bowl. In a separate smaller bowl, add the peanut butter then throw it in the microwave for 30 seconds or until fully melted. Once fully melted, drizzle the peanut butter onto the Chex and stir until completely coated. Next drizzle on raw honey, if the honey is solid throw it in the microwave for 15-30 seconds. Lastly, sprinkle on $\frac{1}{2}$ of the amount of icing sugar, stir, then add the rest of the amount. Let stand for 1-2 minutes then bon appetit!

Nutri Tip: To avoid breaking the Chex I advise using a spatula for stirring.

Nutri's Famous Turkey Meatballs

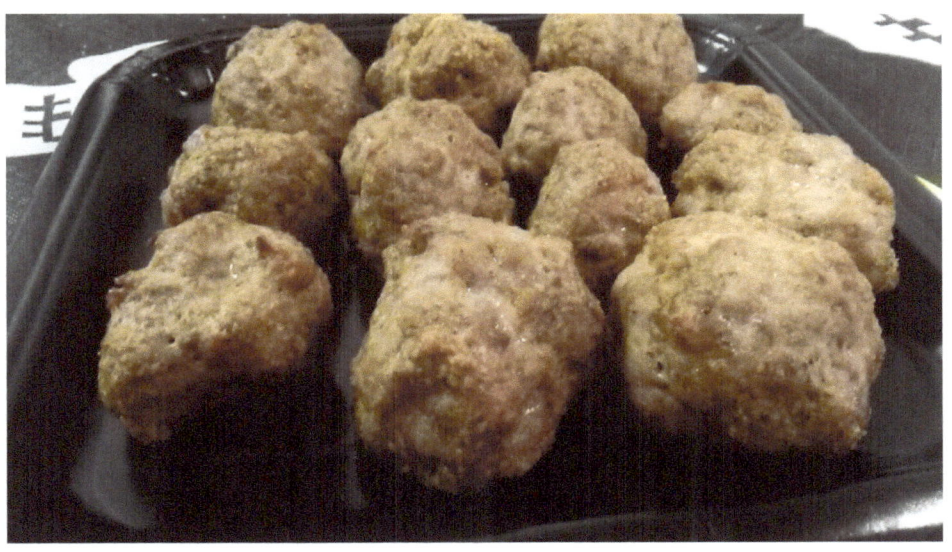

These are an absolute favourite in my home. They are so simple yet so flavorful and so healthy!

You will need:
- **Ground Turkey** (1 pound, raw, makes 12 meatballs)
- **Shake n' Bake Crispy Italian** or Italian bread crumbs ($\frac{1}{2}$ cup)
- **Himalayan Pink Salt** (few pinches)
- **Pepper** (Black or a medley, few pinches)

First preheat your oven to 450 degrees Fahrenheit. Put ground turkey into a large bowl then pour in Shake n' Bake. Lastly add in the salt and pepper, then mix it together with your hands until completely combined. Form into balls and place on a baking sheet lined with aluminum foil.

Throw them in the oven for 15 minutes or until internal temperature is 165 degrees Fahrenheit. Once they are fully cooked plate them and bon appetit!

Nutri Tip: These are great to dip in pretty much anything, but my favourites are marinara or BBQ sauce.

Easy Oven Roasted Whole Chicken

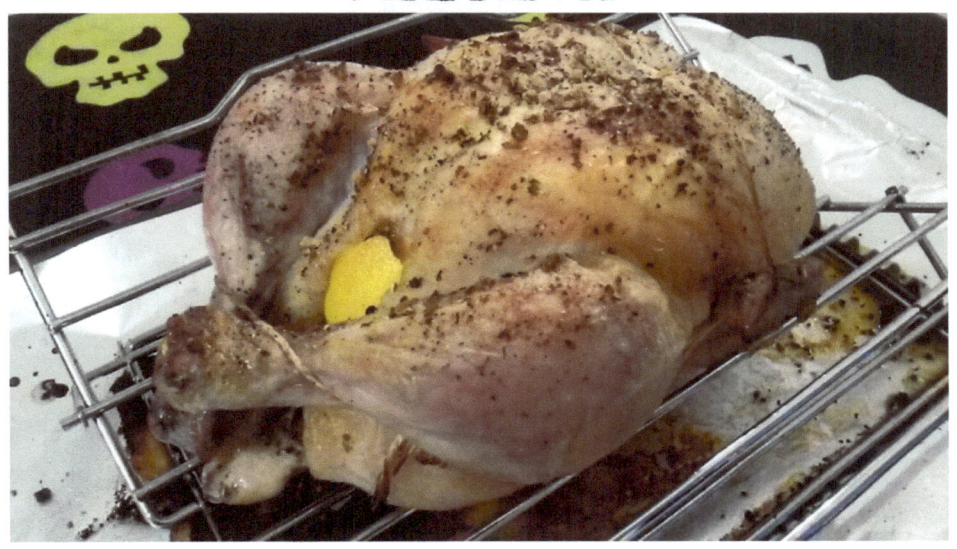

I make this at least once a month! It's the perfect way to get lots of leftovers to pre-portion meals for the month. Saves time and money!

You will need:
- **Whole Chicken** (3 pounds)
- **Lemon** (1, cut into wedges)
- **Orange/Lime** (1, cut into wedges)
- **Black Pepper/Peppercorn Medley** (desired amount)
- **Himalayan Pink Salt** (desired amount)

First preheat your oven to 350 degrees Fahrenheit. Grab a baking sheet covered in aluminum foil or a roasting pan and place the chicken inside. If using a roasting pan, place the whole chicken on top of vegetables so it doesn't touch the bottom. However if using a baking sheet use a wire roasting rack.

Next stuff the cavity of your chicken with as many of the lemon and orange wedges as you can. Dry rub or sprinkle on the salt and pepper then throw it in the oven. Add 20 minutes for every pound the chicken weighs. For example, for this recipe the chicken is 3 pounds so it will be cooked for 1 hour (20min x 3lbs = 60 minutes).

Once out of the oven, using a meat thermometer make sure the chicken reaches an internal temperature of 165 degrees Fahrenheit. To properly measure the chickens temperature, poke the thermometer into the inner thigh without touching bone. If the chicken is fully cooked, time to plate and bon appetit!

Nutri Tip: My favourite ways to use the leftover chicken is for chicken fried rice, chicken chow mein or in my chicken tarts!

English Muffin Pizzas

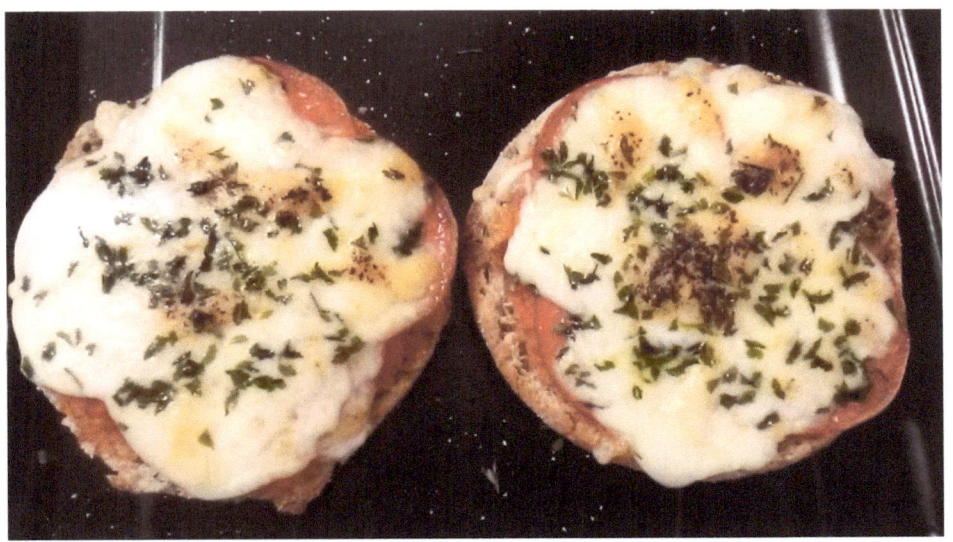

Who doesn't love pizza? This is a way
healthier version though. These are so
quick and easy to make. They make the
perfect portion controlled snack or
lunch!

You will need:
- **English Muffins** (whole wheat)
- **Marinara Sauce** (All Natural)
- **Mozzarella Cheese** (Shredded)
- **Turkey Pepperoni**
- **Dried Parsley**
- **Garlic Powder**
- **Extra Virgin Olive Oil**

First preheat your oven to 375 degrees Fahrenheit. Slice your english muffin in half and drizzle on a small amount of olive oil on each half. Scoop and spread the marinara sauce onto each side of the muffin with a spoon. Next throw on desired amount of pepperoni then sprinkle the shredded mozzarella on top. Lastly sprinkle the parsley and garlic powder on top. Place in the oven on top rack for 2 minutes then broil the tops of the pizzas for another 2 minutes to brown the cheese. Using tongs, remove from oven and let cool for 2 minutes. Once cooled they are ready to eat! Bon appetit!

Nutri Tip: For variety switch up your toppings. My favourite topping to add is orange bell peppers!

Zingy Air fried Turkey Burgers

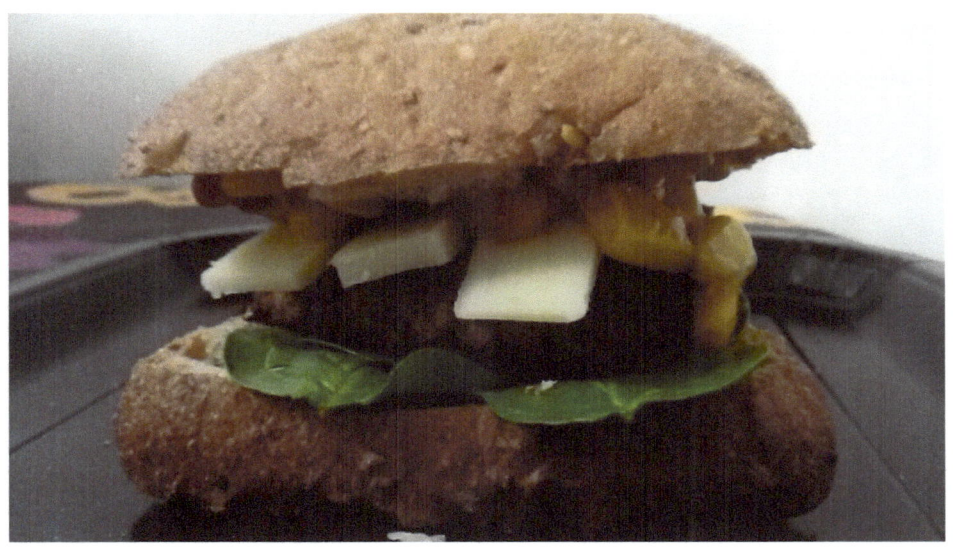

You would skip any burger joint for this healthy gourmet burger. It's so simple and flavorful, you would never think it was healthy!

You will need:
- **Ground Turkey** (1 pound)
- **Ciabatta Buns** (whole wheat or 5 grain)
- **Italian Dressing** (2 tbsp)
- **Mozzarella Cheese** (sliced, desired amount)
- **Corn Salsa** (desired amount)
- **Baby Spinach** (fresh, desired amount)
- **Himalayan Pink Salt** (few pinches)
- **Black Peppercorn** (few pinches)
- **Dried Parsley** (desired amount)
- **Garlic Powder** (desired amount)

First grab a large bowl and throw in the ground turkey. Spoon in the Italian dressing. Next add the herbs and spices. With your hands combine all the ingredients together. Once completely combined use your hands or a manual patty maker. Place patties into the air fryer and cook until desired doneness (for a T-Fal Acti-Fry place burgers in bottom tray).
While burgers are cooking set up your bun with cheese, salsa and spinach. When burgers are cooked place a patty onto your bun, put it together and it's ready to eat! Bon appetit!

Nutri Tip: I choose to make these in the air fryer but you could also make these on a BBQ, a grill, anything!

Strawberry Dream Boats

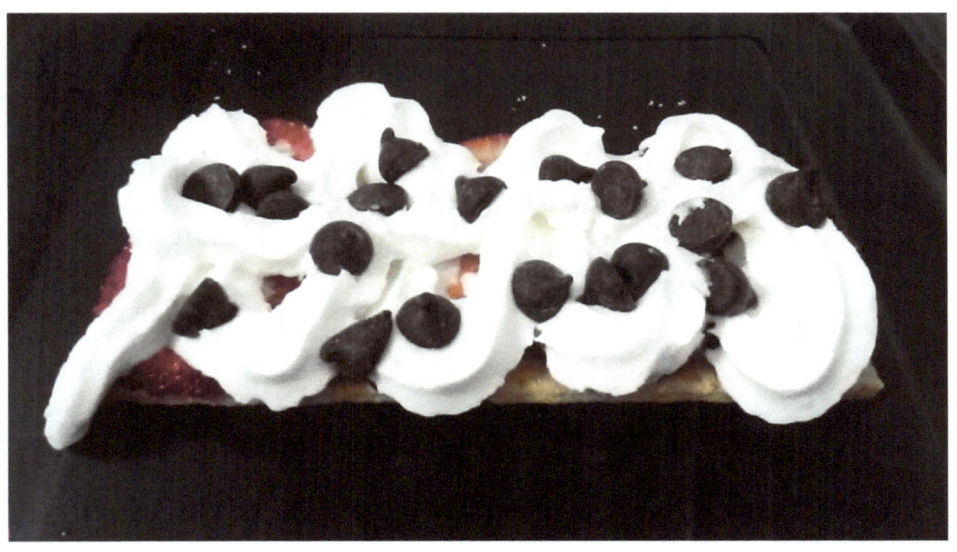

This dessert tastes like a sin but everything about is healthy. It's so easy to make, you can literally whip it up anytime you got a sweet tooth!

You will need:

-**Real Whipped Cream** (aerosol or homemade if desired)
-**Dark Chocolate Chips** (desired amount)
-**Strawberries** (1 strawberry per graham cracker)
-**Graham Crackers** (desired amount)

First slice desired amount of strawberries into slices. Lay down your graham cracker and place the sliced strawberries on top. If using aerosol whipped cream, spray from left to right on top of the strawberries until completely covered. Sprinkle desired amount of dark chocolate chips on top of the whipped cream. Time to take a bite and bon appetit!

Nutri Tip: These are addicting but in a good way. The best part? They're nothing to feel guilty about!

BBQ Chicken Tarts

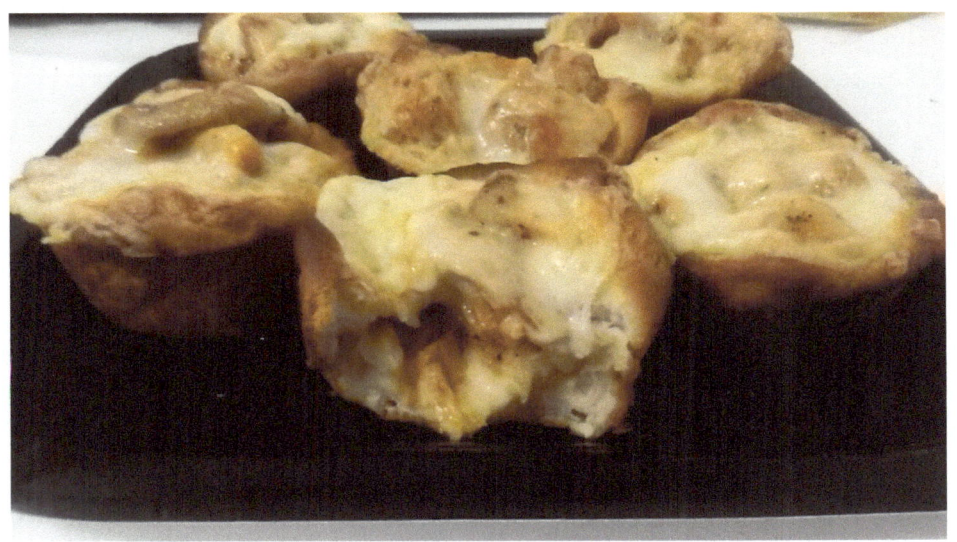

These are great as a pre/post workout snack. It's packed with protein and easy to make anytime!

You will need:
-**Chicken Breasts** (1 pound, cooked and quartered)
-**BBQ** (2-3 tbsp, desired flavor or brand)
-**Dough** (store bought pre-made or homemade)
-**Mozzarella Cheese** (2-3 cups, shredded)

Optional:
-**Parsley** (desired amount)
-**Black Pepper** (desired amount)

First preheat your oven to 400 degrees Fahrenheit. Grab a small bowl and throw in your chicken. Pour the barbecue sauce on top then stir until completely combined.
Next grab a muffin pan and spray it with cooking spray or grease with light butter. Flatten each piece of dough with your hands then place into muffin pan. Try to make them into cups the best you can. Scoop chicken mixture into dough cups then sprinkle shredded cheese on top. Lastly place them in the oven for 10-15 minutes or until golden brown. You can also broil the tops for 2 minutes if desired. Once they are completely cooked, plate and bon appetit!

Nutri Tip: The best part about these is that you can switch up the ingredients for variety, like substitute BBQ for your favourite sauce or even switch up chicken for beef/pork. The options are endless! You can also store these in a Ziploc bag in the refrigerator for up to 3 days.

Ham & Corn Breakfast Bake

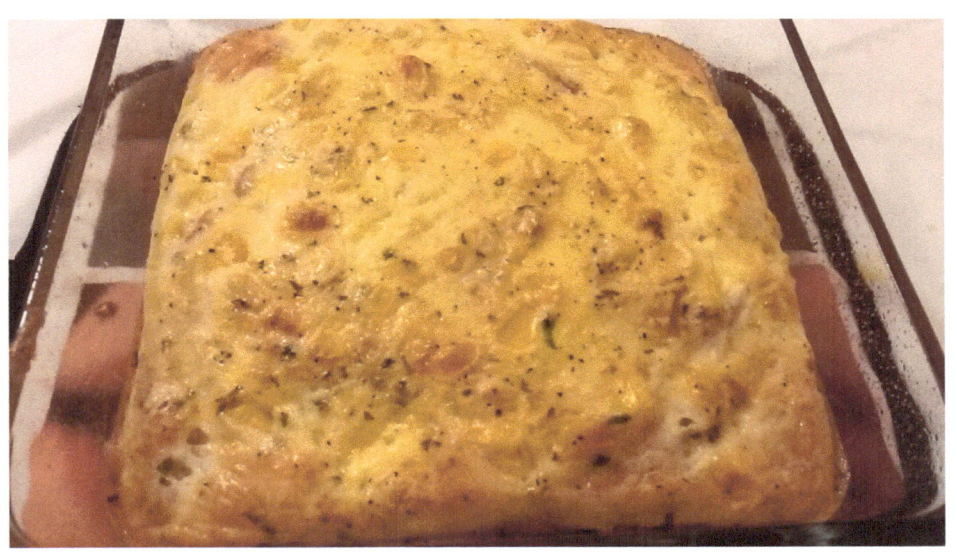

This is such an easy way to get a complete breakfast quick. It also has my favourite vegetable, corn!

You will need:
- **Eggs** (4, brown/white, free run)
- **Mozzarella Cheese** (1 cup, shredded)
- **Ham** (cooked, sliced lunch-meat style, desired flavor)
- **Corn** (1 cup, frozen or fresh)
- **Himalayan Pink Salt** (desired amount)
- **Black Pepper** (desired amount)
- **Parsley** (desired amount)

First preheat your oven to 375 degrees Fahrenheit then grab a 6x6 or any medium sized cake pan. Spray it with cooking spray or grease it with light butter. Dice desired amount of sliced ham. In a large bowl combine all the ingredients except for the corn and stir. Once eggs are completely scrambled, pour mixture into pan. Lastly sprinkle corn onto mixture, then lightly spread with the bottom of a spoon to evenly reach all sides/corners. Place it in the oven for 20 minutes or until eggs are completely set and cooked. Once it's done, plate and bon appetit!

Nutri Tip: I love this recipe because you can grab yourself a piece, throw it in the microwave for 2 minutes and *boom* a quick breakfast! You can also store it in the refrigerator, covered for up to 3 days.

Nutri HBC's Birthday Drink

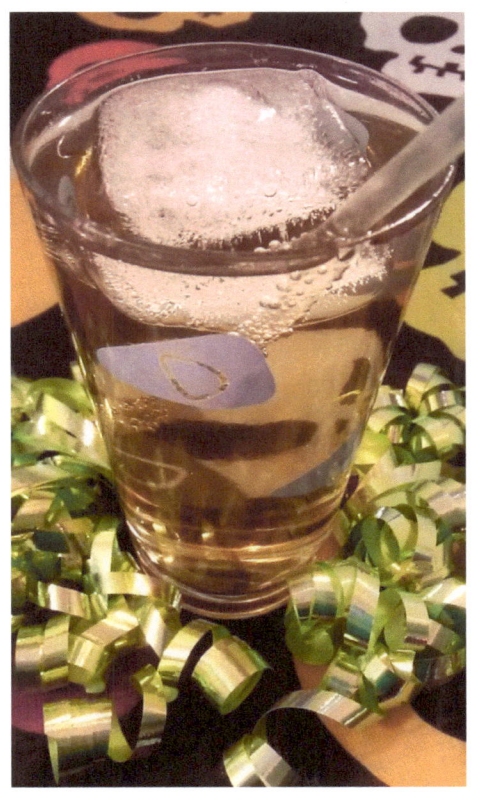

This drink is dedicated to the first year of Nutri HBC. Happy Birthday and to many more nutritious years!

You will need:
-**Ginger ale** (1 part)
-**100% Apple Juice** (1 part)
-**Whisky** (1 ounce, desired brand)
-**Sour Green Apple liqueur** (1 ounce, desired brand)

Optional:
-**Green apple** (1, quartered for garnish)

First grab a highball glass and add desired amount of ice cubes. Add whisky and apple liqueur, in that order. Pour 1 part apple juice then fill the rest of the glass with ginger ale. Add apple for garnish and a straw if desired. Time to party! Cheers!

Nutri Tip: This drink is delicious and it's easy to drink more than one. Just a warning!

Index

Find Me Online

For everything Nutri HBC visit my website

www.nutrihbc.com

Instagram @nutrihbc
Facebook @nutrihbc